Step-by-Step
Plant Based Diet Recipes

Lose Weight Quickly with a Step-by-Step
Plant-Based Diet Recipes Guide. Delicious
Healthy Eating Food, Easy to Prepare!

John Becker

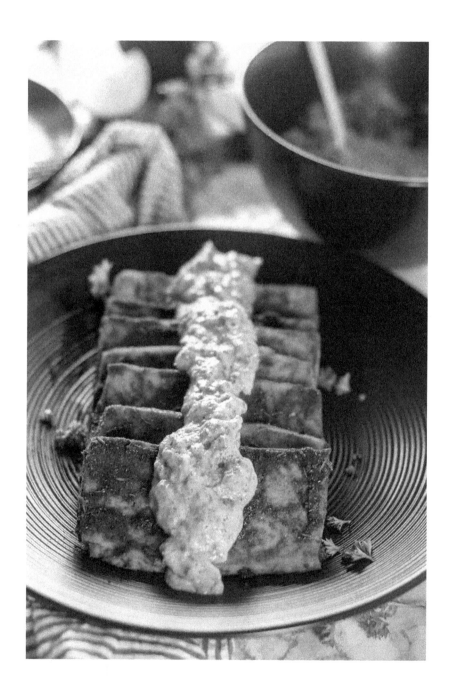

Table of Contents

Introduction

A plant-based diet is a diet based primarily on whole plant foods. It is identical to the regular diet we're used to already, except that it leaves out foods that are not exclusively from plants. Hence, a plant-based diet does away with all types of animal-sourced foods, hydrogenated oils, refined sugars, and processed foods. A whole food plant-based diet comprises not just fruits and vegetables; it also consists of unprocessed or barely-processed oils with healthy monounsaturated fats (like extra-virgin olive oil), whole grains, legumes (essentially lentils and beans), seeds and nuts, as well as herbs and spices.

What makes a plant-based meal (or any meal) fun is the manner with which you make them; the seasoning process; and the combination process that contributes to a fantastic flavor and makes every meal unique and enjoyable. There are lots of delicious recipes (all plant-centered), which will prove helpful in when you intend making mouthwatering, healthy plant-based dishes for personal or household consumption. Provided you're eating these plant-based foods regularly, you'll have very problems with fat or diseases that result from bad dietary habits, and there would be no need for excessive calorie tracking.

Plant-based diet recipes are versatile; they range from colorful Salads to Lentil Stews, and Bean Burritos. The recipes also draw influences from around the globe, with Mexican, Chinese, European, Indian cuisines all part of the vast array of plant-based recipes available to choose from. Why You Ought to Reduce Your Intake of Processed and Animal-Based Foods. You have likely heard over and over that processed food has adverse effects on your health. You might have also been told repeatedly to stay away from foods with lots of preservatives; nevertheless, nobody ever offered any genuine or concrete facts about why you ought to avoid these foods and why they are unsafe. Consequently, let us properly dissect it to help you properly comprehend why you ought to stay away from these healthy eating offenders. They have massive habit-forming characteristics. Humans have a predisposition towards being addicted to some specific foods; however, the reality is that the fault is not wholly ours. Every one of the unhealthy treats we relish now and then triggers the dopamine release in our brains. This creates a pleasurable effect in our brain, but the excitement is usually short-lived. The discharged dopamine additionally causes an attachment connection gradually, and this is the reason some people consistently go back to eat certain unhealthy foods even when they know it's unhealthy and unnecessary. You can get rid of this by taking out that inducement completely. They are sugar-laden and plenteous in glucose-fructose syrup. Animal-based and processed foods are laden with refined sugars and glucose-fructose syrup which has almost no beneficial food nutrient. An ever-increasing number of studies are affirming what several people presumed from the start; that genetically modified foods bring about inflammatory bowel disease, which consequently makes it increasingly difficult for the body to assimilate essential nutrients. The disadvantages that result from your body being unable to assimilate essential nutrients from consumed foods rightly cannot be overemphasized. Processed and animal-based food products contain plenteous amounts of refined carbohydrates. Indeed, your body requires carbohydrates to give it the needed energy to run body capacities. In any case, refining carbs dispenses with the fundamental supplements; in the way that refining entire grains disposes of the whole grain part. What remains, in the wake of refining, is what's considered as empty carbs or empty calories. These can negatively affect the metabolic system in your body by sharply increasing your blood sugar and insulin quantities. They contain lots of synthetic ingredients. At the point when your body is taking in non-natural ingredients, it regards them as foreign substances. Your body treats them as a health threat. Your body isn't accustomed to identifying synthetic compounds like sucralose or these synthesized sugars. Hence, in defense of your health against this foreign "aggressor," your body does what it's capable of to safeguard your health. It sets off an immune reaction to tackle this "enemy" compound, which indirectly weakens your body's general disease alertness, making you susceptible to illnesses. The concentration and energy expended by your body in ensuring your immune system remain safe could instead be devoted somewhere else. They contain constituent elements that set off an excitable reward sensation in your body. A part of processed and animal-based foods contain compounds like glucose-fructose syrup, monosodium glutamate, and specific food dyes that can trigger some addiction. They rouse your body to receive a benefit in return whenever you consume them. Monosodium glutamate, for example, is added to many store-bought baked foods. This additive slowly conditions your palates to relish the taste. It gets mental just by how your brain interrelates with your taste sensors.

This reward-centric arrangement makes you crave it increasingly, which ends up exposing you to the danger of over consuming calories.

For animal protein, usually, the expression "subpar" is used to allude to plant proteins since they generally have lower levels of essential amino acids as against animal-sourced protein. Nevertheless, what the vast majority don't know is that large amounts of essential amino acids can prove detrimental to your health. Let me break it down further for you.

Baked Okra and Tomato

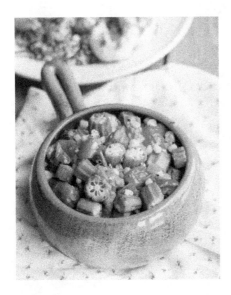

Preparation Time: 10 minutes

Cooking Time: 75 minutes

Servings: 6

Ingredients:

> ½ cup lima beans, frozen
>
> 4 tomatoes, chopped
>
> 8 ounces okra, fresh and washed, stemmed, sliced into
> > ½ inch thick slices
>
> 1 onion, sliced into rings
>
> ½ sweet pepper, seeded and sliced thin
>
> Pinch of crushed red pepper
>
> Salt to taste

Directions:

Preheat your oven to 350 degrees Fahrenheit

Cook lima beans in water accordingly and drain them, take a 2quart casserole tin

Add all listed ingredients to the dish and cover with foil, bake for 45 minutes

Uncover the dish, stir well and bake for 35 minutes more

Stir then serve, and enjoy!

Nutrition:

Calories: 55

Fat: 0g

Carbohydrates: 12g

Protein: 3g

Curried Apple

Preparation Time: 10 minutes

Cooking Time: 90 minutes

Servings: 4

Ingredients:

> 1 tablespoon fresh lemon juice
>
> ½ cup of water
>
> 2 apples, Fuji or Honeycrisp, cored and thinly sliced into rings
>
> 1 teaspoon curry powder

Directions:

> Set the oven to 200F, take a rimmed baking sheet and line with parchment paper
>
> Take a bowl and mix in lemon juice and water, add apples and soak for 2 minutes
>
> Pat them dry and arrange in a single layer on your baking sheet, dust curry powder on top of apple slices
>
> Bake for 45 minutes. After 45 minutes, turn the apples and bake for 45 minutes more
>
> Let them cool for extra crispiness, serve and enjoy!

Nutrition:

Calories: 240

Fat: 13g

Carbohydrates: 20g

Protein: 6g

Grilled Eggplant Steaks

Preparation Time: 10 minutes

Cooking Time: 10 minutes

Servings: 4

Ingredients:

> 4 Roma tomatoes, diced
>
> 8 ounces cashew cream
>
> 2 eggplants
>
> 1 tablespoon olive oil
>
> 1 cup parsley, chopped
>
> 1 cucumber, diced
>
> Salt and pepper to taste

Directions:

> Slice eggplants into three thick steaks, drizzle with oil, and season with salt and pepper
>
> Grill in a pan for 4 minutes per side
>
> Top with remaining ingredients
>
> Serve and enjoy!

Nutrition:

Calories: 86

Fat: 7g

Carbohydrates: 12g

Protein: 8g

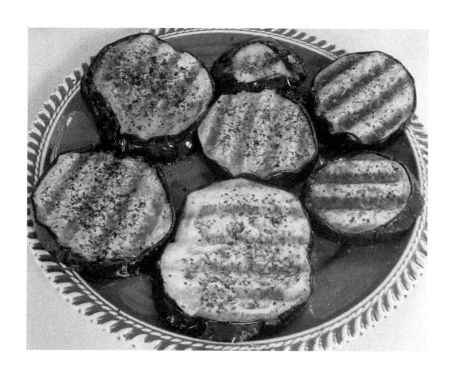

Glazed Avocado

Preparation Time: 10 minutes

Cooking Time: 12 minutes

Servings: 4

Ingredients:

- 1 tablespoon stevia
- 1 teaspoon olive oil
- 1 teaspoon water
- 1 teaspoon lemon juice
- ½ teaspoon rosemary, dried
- ½ teaspoon ground black pepper
- 2 avocados, peeled, pitted and cut into large pieces

Directions:

1. Heat up a pan with the oil over medium heat, add the avocados, stevia and the other ingredients, toss, cook for 12 minutes, divide into bowls and serve.

Nutrition:

Calories 262,Fat 9.6,Fiber 0.1,Carbs 6.5,Protein 7.9

Mango and Leeks balls

Preparation Time: 20 minutes

Cooking Time: 10 minutes

Servings: 4

Ingredients:

- 1 tablespoon mango puree
- 1 cup leeks, chopped
- ½ cup tofu, crumbled
- 1 teaspoon dried oregano
- 1 tablespoon almond flour
- 1 teaspoon olive oil
- 1 tablespoon flax meal
- ½ teaspoon chili flakes

Directions:

2. In the mixing bowl, mix up mango puree with leeks, tofu and the other ingredients except the oil and stir well.
3. Make the small balls.
4. After this, pour the olive oil in the skillet and heat it up.
5. Add the balls in the skillet and cook them for 4 minutes from each side.

Nutrition:

Calories 147

Fat 8.6

Fiber 4.5

Carbs 5.6

Protein 5.3

Spicy Carrots and Olives

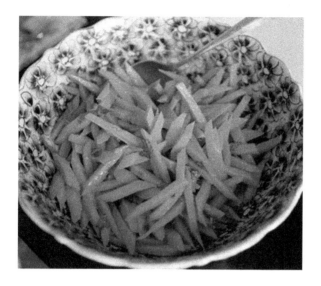

Preparation Time: 15 minutes

Cooking Time: 10 minutes

Servings: 4

Ingredients:

½ teaspoon hot paprika

1 red chili pepper, minced

¼ teaspoon ground cumin

¼ teaspoon dried oregano

¼ teaspoon dried basil

½ teaspoon salt

1 tablespoon olive oil

1 pound baby carrots, peeled

1 cup kalamata olives, pitted and halved

Juice of 1 lime

Directions:

Heat up a pan with the oil over medium heat, add the carrots, olives and the other ingredients, toss, cook for 10 minutes, divide between plates and serve.

Nutrition:

Calories 141

Fat 5.8

Fiber 4.3

Carbs 7.5

Protein 9.6

Harissa Mushrooms

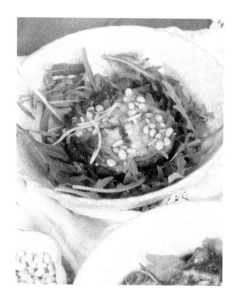

Preparation Time: 15 minutes

Cooking Time: 30 minutes

Servings: 4

Ingredients:

    1-pound mushroom caps

    1 teaspoon harissa

    1 teaspoon rosemary, dried

    2 spring onions, chopped

    1 leek, sliced

    1 teaspoon thyme, dried

    1 cup crushed tomatoes

    1 teaspoon sweet paprika

A pinch of salt and black pepper

1 tablespoon olive oil

½ teaspoon lemon juice

Directions:

In a roasting pan, mix the mushrooms with the harissa,
rosemary and the other ingredients and toss.
Preheat the oven to 360F and put the pan inside.
Cook the mix for 30 minutes, divide between plates
and serve.

Nutrition:

Calories 250

Fat 12.1

Fiber 5.3

Carbs 14.5

Protein 12.9

Leeks and Artichokes Mix

Preparation Time: 10 minutes

Cooking Time: 30 minutes

Servings: 4

Ingredients:

2 cups canned artichoke hearts, drained and quartered

3 leeks, sliced

1 cup cherry tomatoes, halved

¼ cup coconut cream

1 tablespoon almond flakes

1 teaspoon olive oil

1 teaspoon oregano, dried

1 teaspoon salt

1 teaspoon ground black pepper

¼ cup of chives, chopped

Directions:

Heat up a pan with the oil over medium heat, add the leeks, oregano, salt and pepper, stir and cook for 10 minutes.

Add artichokes and the other ingredients, toss, cook for 20 minutes, divide into bowls and serve.

Nutrition:

Calories 234

Fat 9.7

Fiber 4.2

Carbs 9.6

Protein 12.3

Coconut Avocado

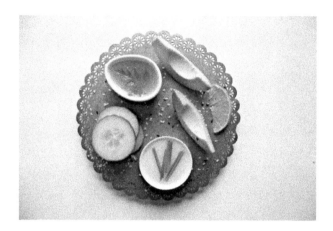

Preparation Time: 10 minutes

Cooking Time: 0 minutes

Servings: 2

Ingredients:

2 avocados, halved, pitted and roughly cubed

1 teaspoon dried thyme

2 tablespoons coconut cream

1 cup spring onions, chopped

1 teaspoon turmeric powder

Salt and black pepper to the taste

¼ teaspoon cayenne pepper

½ teaspoon onion powder

½ teaspoon garlic powder

1 teaspoon paprika

Salt and black pepper to the taste

2 tablespoons lemon juice

Directions:

In a bowl, mix the avocados with the thyme, coconut cream and the other ingredients, toss, divide between plates and serve.

Nutrition:
Calories 160

Fat 6.9

Fiber 7

Carbs 12

Protein 7

Avocado Cream

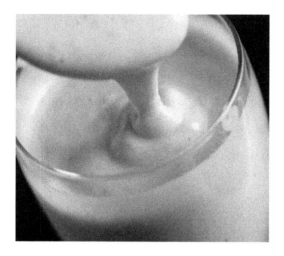

Preparation Time: 10 minutes

Cooking Time: 0 minutes

Servings: 4

Ingredients:

2 avocados, pitted, peeled and chopped

3 cups veggie stock

1 teaspoon curry powder

1 teaspoon cumin, ground

1 teaspoon basil, dried

2 scallions, chopped

Salt and black pepper to the taste

2 tablespoons coconut oil

2/3 cup coconut cream, unsweetened

Directions:

In a blender, mix the avocados with the stock, curry powder and the other ingredients, blend and serve.

Nutrition:

Calories 212,Fat 8,Fiber 4,Carbs 6.1,Protein 4.1

Tamarind Avocado Bowls

Preparation Time: 10 minutes

Cooking Time: 0 minutes

Servings: 2

Ingredients:

- 1 teaspoon cumin seeds
- 1 tablespoon olive oil
- ½ teaspoon garam masala
- 1 teaspoon ground ginger
- 2 avocados, peeled, pitted and roughly cubed
- 1 mango, peeled, and cubed
- 1 cup cherry tomatoes, halved
- ½ teaspoon cayenne pepper
- 1 teaspoon turmeric powder
- 3 tablespoons tamarind paste

Directions:

In a bowl, mix the avocados with the mango and the other ingredients, toss and serve.

Nutrition:

Calories 170,Fat 4.5,Fiber 3,Carbs 5,Protein 6

Onion and Tomato Bowls

Preparation Time: 10 minutes

Cooking Time: 0 minutes

Servings: 4

Ingredients:

> 1 tablespoon olive oil
>
> 2 red bell peppers, cut into thin strips
>
> 2 red onions, cut into thin strips
>
> Salt and black pepper to the taste
>
> 1 teaspoon dried basil
>
> 1 pound tomatoes, cut into wedges
>
> 1 teaspoon balsamic vinegar
>
> 1 teaspoon sweet paprika

Directions:

> In a bowl, mix the peppers with the onions and the other ingredients, toss and serve.

Nutrition:

Calories 107

Fat 4.5

Fiber 2

Carbs 7.1

Protein 6

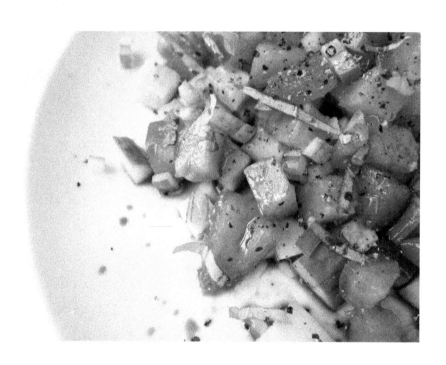

Avocado and Leeks Mix

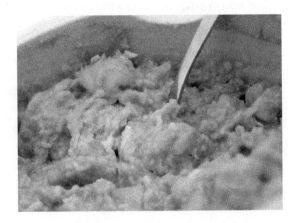

Preparation Time: 10 minutes

Cooking Time: 0 minutes

Servings: 4

Ingredients:

> 1 small red onion, chopped
>
> 2 avocados, pitted, peeled and chopped
>
> 1 teaspoon chili powder
>
> 2 leeks, sliced
>
> 1 cup cucumber, cubed
>
> 1 cup cherry tomatoes, halved
>
> Salt and black pepper to the taste
>
> 2 tablespoons cumin powder
>
> 2 tablespoons lime juice
>
> 1 tablespoon parsley, chopped

Directions:

In a bowl, mix the onion with the avocados, chili powder and the other ingredients, toss and serve.

Nutrition:

Calories 120,Fat 2,Fiber 2,Carbs 7,Protein 4

Lemon Lentils and Carrots

Preparation Time: 10 minutes

Cooking Time: 20 minutes

Servings: 6

Ingredients:

> 1 cup brown lentils, soaked overnight and drained
>
> 1 cup carrots, shredded
>
> 1 cup spring onions, chopped
>
> 1 teaspoon curry powder
>
> 1 teaspoon turmeric powder
>
> 1 teaspoon garam masala
>
> 2 tablespoons lemon juice
>
> ¼ cup parsley, chopped
>
> 2 garlic cloves, minced
>
> A pinch of salt and black pepper
>
> ½ teaspoon thyme, dried
>
> 2 tablespoons olive oil

Directions:

> Heat up a pan with the oil over medium heat, add the garlic, carrots and spring onions and cook for 5 minutes.
>
> Add the lentils and the other ingredients, toss and simmer over medium heat for 15 minutes.

Divide between plates and serve.

Nutrition:

Calories 240

Fat 7

Fiber 3.4

Carbs 12

Protein 6

Cabbage Bowls

Preparation Time: 10 minutes

Cooking Time: 10 minutes

Servings: 4

Ingredients:

> 1 green cabbage head, shredded
>
> 1 red cabbage head, shredded
>
> 1 teaspoon garam masala
>
> 1 teaspoon basil, dried
>
> 1 teaspoon coriander, ground
>
> 1 teaspoon mustard seeds
>
> 1 tablespoon balsamic vinegar
>
> ¼ cup tomatoes, crushed
>
> A pinch of salt and black pepper
>
> 3 carrots, shredded
>
> 1 yellow bell pepper, chopped
>
> 1 orange bell pepper, chopped
>
> 1 red bell pepper, chopped
>
> 2 tablespoons dill, chopped
>
> 2 tablespoons olive oil

Directions:

> Heat up a pan with the oil over medium heat, add the peppers and carrots and cook for 2 minutes.

Add the cabbage and the other ingredients, toss, cook for 10 minutes, divide between plates and serve.

Nutrition:

Calories 150

Fat 9

Fiber 4

Carbs 3.3

Protein 4.4

Pomegranate and Pears Salad

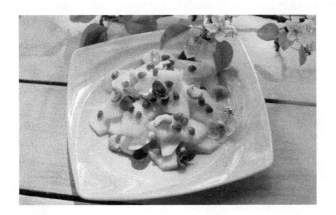

Preparation Time: 10 minutes

Cooking Time: 0 minutes

Servings: 3

Ingredients:

  3 big pears, cored and cut with a spiralizer

  ¾ cup pomegranate seeds

  2 cups baby spinach

  ½ cup black olives, pitted and cubed

  ¾ cup walnuts, chopped1 tablespoon olive oil

  1 tablespoon coconut sugar

  1 teaspoon white sesame seeds

  2 tablespoons chives, chopped

  1 tablespoon balsamic vinegar

  1 garlic clove, minced

  A pinch of sea salt and black pepper

Directions:

In a bowl, mix the pears with the pomegranate seeds, spinach and the other ingredients, toss and serve.

Nutrition:

Calories 200

Fat 3.9

Fiber 4

Carbs 6

Protein 3.3

Bulgur and Tomato Mix

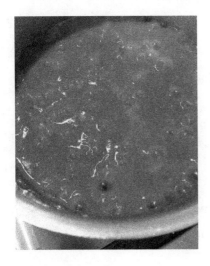

Preparation Time: 15 minutes

Cooking Time: 0 minutes

Servings: 4

Ingredients:

> 1 ½ cups hot water
>
> 1 cup bulgur
>
> Juice of 1 lime
>
> 1 cup cherry tomatoes, halved
>
> 4 tablespoons cilantro, chopped
>
> ½ cup cranberries, dried
>
> Juice of ½ lemon
>
> 1 teaspoon oregano, dried
>
> 1/3 cup almonds, sliced

¼ cup green onions, chopped

½ cup red bell peppers, chopped

½ cup carrots, grated

1 tablespoon avocado oil

A pinch of sea salt and black pepper

Directions:

Place bulgur into a bowl, add boiling water to it, stir,
cover and set aside for 15 minutes.

Fluff bulgur with a fork and transfer to a bowl.

Add the rest of the ingredients, toss and serve.

Nutrition:

Calories 260

Fat 4.4

Fiber 3

Carbs 7

Protein 10

Beans Mix

Preparation Time: 10 minutes

Cooking Time: 15 minutes

Servings: 4

Ingredients:

- 1 ½ cups cooked black beans
- 1 cup cooked red kidney beans
- ½ teaspoon garlic powder
- ½ teaspoon smoked paprika
- 2 teaspoons chili powder
- 1 tablespoon olive oil
- 1 ½ cups chickpeas, cooked
- 1 teaspoon garam masala
- 1 red bell pepper, chopped
- 2 tomatoes, chopped
- 1 cup cashews, chopped
- ½ cup veggie stock
- 1 tablespoon balsamic vinegar
- 1 tablespoon oregano, chopped
- 1 tablespoon dill, chopped
- 1 cup corn kernels, chopped

Directions:

Heat up a pan with the oil over medium heat, add the beans, garlic powder, chili powder and the other ingredients, toss and cook for 15 minutes.

Divide between plates and serve.

Nutrition:

Calories 300

Fat 8.3

Fiber 3.3

Carbs 6

Protein 13

Flavorful Refried Beans

Preparation Time: 15 Minutes

Cooking Time: 8 hours

Servings: 8

Ingredients:

- 3 cups of pinto beans, rinsed

- 1 small jalapeno pepper, seeded and chopped

- 1 medium-sized white onion, peeled and sliced

- 2 tablespoons of minced garlic

- 5 teaspoons of salt

- 2 teaspoons of ground black pepper

- 1/4 teaspoon of ground cumin

- 9 cups of water

Directions:

1. Using a 6-quarts slow cooker, place all the **Ingredients:** and stir until it mixes properly.

2. Cover the top, plug in the slow cooker; adjust the cooking time to 6 hours, let it cook on high heat setting and add more water if the beans get too dry.

3. When the beans are done, drain them and reserve the liquid.

4. Mash the beans using a potato masher and pour in the reserved cooking liquid until it reaches your desired mixture.

5. Serve immediately.

Nutrition:

Calories: 198

Carbs: 22g

Fat: 7g

Protein: 19g

Quinoa Enchiladas

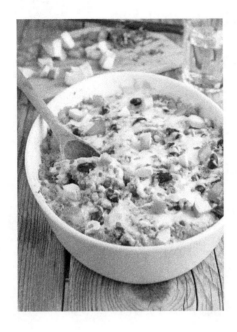

Preparation time: 10 minutes

Cooking time: 40 minutes

Servings: 2

Ingredients:

- 1 tablespoon coconut oil

- 2 cloves garlic, minced

- 1 small yellow onion, chopped

- 3/4 pounds baby bella mushrooms, chopped

- 1/2 cup diced green chilis

- 1/2 teaspoon ground cumin

- 1/4 teaspoon sea salt (or to taste)

- 1 can organic, low sodium black beans or 1-1/2 cup cooked black beans

- 1-1/2 cup cooked quinoa

- 10 6-inch corn tortillas

- 1-1/4 cup organic, low sodium tomato or enchilada sauce

Directions:

1. Preheat oven to 350 degrees.

2. Heat coconut oil in a large pot over medium heat.

3. Sautee onion and garlic till onion is translucent (about 5-8 min) and add mushrooms and cook until liquid has been released and evaporated (another 5 min).

4. Add the chilis to the pot and give them a stir for 2 minutes.

5. Add the cumin, sea salt, black beans and quinoa, and continue heating the mixture until it's completely warm.

6. Spread a thin layer (1/2 cup) of marinara or enchilada sauce in the bottom of a casserole dish.

7. Place a third of a cup of quinoa mixture in the center of a corn tortilla and roll it up. Place the tortilla, seam down, in the casserole dish.

8. Repeat with all remaining tortillas and then cover them with 3/4 cup of additional sauce.

9. Bake for 25 minutes, and serve.

Nutrition:

Calories: 201, Carbs: 4g, Fat: 4g ,Protein: 11g

October Potato Soup

Preparation time: 5 minutes

Cooking time: 20 minutes

Servings: 3

Ingredients:

- 4 minced garlic cloves

- 2 teaspoon coconut oil

- 3 diced celery stalks

- 1 diced onion

- 2 teaspoon yellow mustard seeds

- 5 diced Yukon potatoes

- 6 cups vegetable broth

- 1 teaspoon oregano

- 1 teaspoon paprika

- 1/2 teaspoon cayenne pepper

- 1 teaspoon chili powder

- Salt and pepper to taste

Directions:

1. Begin by sautéing the garlic and the mustard seeds together in the oil in a large soup pot.

2. Next, add the onion and sauté the mixture for another five minutes.

3. Add the celery, the broth, the potatoes, and all the spices, and continue to stir.

4. Allow the soup to simmer for thirty minutes without a cover.

5. Next, Position about three cups of the soup in a blender, and puree the soup until you've reached a smooth consistency. Pour this back into the big soup pot, stir, and serve warm. Enjoy.

Nutrition:

Calories: 203

Carbs: 12g

Fat: 7g

Protein: 9g

Black Bean and Quinoa Salad with Quick Cumin Dressing

Preparation time: 10 minutes

Cooking time: 35 minutes

Servings: 2

Ingredients:

For the salad:

- 1 cup dry quinoa, rinsed

- Dash salt

- 2 cups vegetable broth or water

- 1/2 large cucumber, diced neatly

- 1 small bell pepper, diced neatly

- 1 can BPA free, organic black beans

- 10-15 basil leaves, chopped into a chiffonade

- 1/4 cup fresh cilantro, chopped

- For the vinaigrette:

- 2 tablespoon extra-virgin olive oil

- 1/4 cup apple cider vinegar

- 1 tablespoon agave or maple syrup

- 1 tablespoon dijon mustard

- 1 teaspoon cumin

- Salt and pepper to taste

Directions:

1. Rinse quinoa through a sieve till the water runs clear and transfer it to a small or medium sized pot.

2. Add two cups of vegetable broth or water and dash of salt.

3. Boil water and then allow simmer. Cover the pot so that the lid is on with a little gap to allow water escape.

4. Simmer till quinoa has absorbed all of the liquid and is fluffy (about 15-20 minutes).

5. Transfer cooked quinoa to a mixing bowl.

6. Add chopped vegetables, black beans, and herbs.

7. Whisk dressing **Ingredients:** and add the dressing to the salad, and serve.

Nutrition:

Calories: 252, Carbs: 5g, Fat: 8g, Protein: 12g

Sweet Potato and Black Bean Chili

Preparation time: 15 minutes

Cooking time: 40 minutes

Servings: 3

Ingredients:

- 1-1/2 cup dried black beans

- 4 cups sweet potato, diced into 3/4 inch cubes

- 1 tablespoon olive oil

- 1-1/2 cups chopped white or yellow onion

- 2 cloves garlic, minced

- 1 chipotle pepper in adobo, chopped finely

- 2 teaspoons cumin powder

- 1/2 teaspoon smoked paprika

- 1 tablespoon ground chili powder

- 1 14 or 15 ounce can of organic, diced tomatoes

- 1 can organic, low sodium black beans (or 1-1/2 cups cooked black beans)

- 2 cups low sodium vegetable broth.

- Sea salt to taste

Directions:

1. Heat the tablespoon of oil in a Dutch oven or a large pot.

2. Sauté the onion for a few minutes, then add the sweet potato and garlic and keep sautéing until the onions are soft for about 8-10 minutes.

3. Add the chili in adobo, the cumin, the chili powder, and the smoked paprika and eat until the spices are very fragrant.

4. Add the tomatoes, black beans, and vegetable broth.

5. When broth is bubbling, reduce to a simmer and cook for approximately 25-30 minutes, or until the sweet potatoes are tender.

6. Add more broth as needed, and season to taste with salt.

Nutrition:

Calories: 232,Carbs: 4g, Fat: 9g, Protein: 13g

Rice with Asparagus and Cauliflower

Preparation time: 5 minutes

Cooking time: 20 minutes

Servings: 2

Ingredients:

- 3 ounces' asparagus

- 3 ounces' cauliflower, chopped

- 2 ounces' tomato sauce

- 1/2 cup of brown rice

- 3/4 cup of water

- 1/3 teaspoon salt

- 1/4 teaspoon ground black pepper

- 1/4 teaspoon garlic powder

- 1 tablespoon olive oil

Directions:

1. Take a medium saucepan, place it over medium heat, add oil, add asparagus and cauliflower and then sauté for 5 to 7 minutes until golden brown.

2. Season with garlic powder, salt, and black pepper, stir in tomato sauce, and then cook for 1 minute.

3. Add rice, pour in water, stir until mixed, cover with a lid and cook for 10 to 12 minutes until rice has absorbed all the liquid and become tender.

4. When done, remove the pan from heat, fluff rice with a fork, and then serve.

Nutrition:

Calories: 257

Carbs: 4g

Fat: 4g

Protein: 40g

Creamy Broccoli Soup

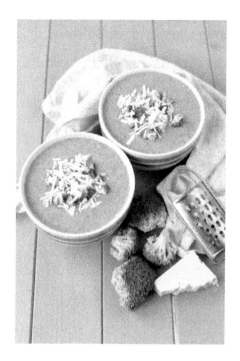

Preparation time: 15 minutes

Cooking time: 30 minutes

Servings: 4

Ingredients:

- 4 cup broccoli florets

- 1/2 teaspoon ground nutmeg

- 1 small avocado, peel and sliced

- 2 cups vegetable broth

Directions:

1. Add broth into the pot and bring to simmer over medium-high heat.

2. Add broccoli into the pot and cook for 8 minutes or until tender.

3. Reduce heat to low and add avocado and nutmeg.

4. Whisk well and cook for 4 minutes.

5. Using blender, puree the soup until smooth.

6. Serve and enjoy.

Nutrition:

Calories: 159

Carbs: 4g

Fat: 4g

Protein: 11g

Crispy Cauliflower

Preparation time: 5 minutes

Cooking time: 15 minutes

Servings: 2

Ingredients:

- 6 ounces of cauliflower florets

- 1/2 of zucchini, sliced

- 1/2 teaspoon of sea salt

- 1/2 tablespoon curry powder

- 1/4 teaspoon maple syrup

- 2 tablespoons olive oil

Directions:

1. Switch on the oven, then set it to 450 degrees F and let it preheat.

2. Meanwhile, take a medium bowl, add cauliflower florets and zucchini slices, add remaining **Ingredients:** reserving 1 tablespoon oil, and toss until well coated.

3. Take a medium skillet pan, place it over medium-high heat, add remaining oil and wait until it gets hot.

4. Spread cauliflower and zucchini in a single layer and sauté for 5 minutes, tossing frequently.

5. Then transfer the pan into the oven and then bake for 8 to 10 minutes until vegetables have turned golden brown and thoroughly cooked, stirring halfway.

Nutrition:

Calories: 161

Carbs: 2g

Fat: 2g

Protein: 7g

Cabbage Zucchini Salad

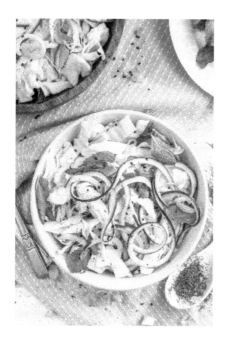

Preparation time: 5 minutes

Cooking time: 10 minutes

Servings: 3

Ingredients:

- 1 medium zucchini, spiralized

- 1 teaspoon stevia

- 1/3 cup rice vinegar

- 3/4 cup olive oil

- 1 cup almonds, sliced

- 1 cup sunflower seeds shelled

- 1 lb cabbage, shredded

Directions:

1. Chop spiralized zucchini into small pieces and set aside.

2. In large mixing bowl, combine together cabbage, almonds, and sunflower seeds

3. Stir in zucchini

4. In a small bowl, mix together oil, stevia, and vinegar. Whisk well and pour over vegetables.

5. Toss salad well and place in refrigerator for 2 hours

6. Serve and enjoy

Nutrition:

Calories: 211

Carbs: 2g

Fat: 3g

Protein: 9g

Black Bean And Corn Burgers

Preparation time: 10 minutes

Cooking time: 15 minutes

Servings: 4

Ingredients:

- 1 tablespoon coconut oil

- 1 small yellow onion, chopped

- 1 cup fresh, frozen or canned organic corn kernels

- 1 can organic, low sodium black beans, drained (or 1-1/2 cups cooked black beans)

- 1 cup brown rice, cooked

- 1/4 cup oat flour (or ground, rolled oats)

- 1/4 cup tomato paste

- 2 teaspoon cumin

- 1 heaping teaspoon paprika

- 1 heaping teaspoon chili powder

- 1/2 - 1 teaspoon sea salt (to taste)

- Black pepper or red pepper, to taste

Directions:

1. Preheat your oven to 350 F.

2. Heat the coconut oil in a large sauté pan and add the onion and saute till onion is golden, soft, and fragrant (about 5-8 minutes).

3. Add corn, beans and tomato paste to the pan and heat through.

4. Place cooked rice into the bowl of a food processor.

5. Add the beans, onion, tomato paste, and corn mixture.

6. Pulse to combine.

7. Add spices, oat flour, and a touch of water, if needed.

8. Pulse more, until you have a thick and sticky (but pliable) mixture.

9. If the mixture is too wet, add a tablespoon or two of additional oat flour.

Nutrition:

Calories: 129

Carbs: 4g

Fat: 2g

Protein: 10g

Creamy Cheese Asparagus

Preparation time: 10 minutes

Cooking time: 20 minutes

Servings: 2

Ingredients:

- 1 lb asparagus, wash and trim off the ends

- 1 cup mozzarella cheese, shredded

- 1/2 cup asiago cheese, grated

- 1 tablespoon Italian seasoning

- 1 cup heavy whipping cream

- Pepper

- Salt

Directions:

1. Preheat the oven to 400F.

2. Spray baking dish with cooking spray and set aside

3. Place asparagus into the prepared baking dish

4. In a small bowl, whisk together heavy cream, asiago cheese, Italian seasoning, pepper and salt.

5. Pour heavy cream mixture over the asparagus.

6. Sprinkle with shredded mozzarella cheese

7. Bake in preheated oven for 18 minutes

Nutrition:

Calories: 163

Carbs: 2g

Fat: 4g

Protein: 8g

Kale Avocado Salad

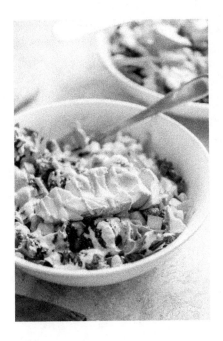

Preparation time: 5 minutes

Cooking time: 20 minutes

Servings: 2

Ingredients:

- 1 Medium avocado, peel and cut into cubes

- 2 tablespoon pine nuts

- 2 tablespoon olive oil

- 1/2 small orange juice

- 1/2 lime juice

- 2 cups kale, chopped

- 1/4 teaspoon black pepper

- 1/2 teaspoon sea salt

Directions:

1. Heat 2-litre water into the pot

2. Add salt and kale into the pot and cool for 10-20 minutes.

3. Drain kale well and set aside to cool

4. Add kale, avocado, and pine nuts into the mixing bowl and toss well.

5. Season salad with pepper and salt

6. In a small bowl, mix together oil, orange juice, and lime juice and pour over salad.

Nutrition:

Calories: 252

Carbs: 4g

Fat: 3g

Protein: 6g

Ginger Lime Chickpea Sweet Potato Burgers

Preparation time: 10 minutes

Cooking time: 40 minutes

Servings: 2

Ingredients:

- 3/4 cup cooked chickpeas

- 1/2 small onion

- 1 inch ginger, chopped

- 1 teaspoon coconut oil

- 1-1/2 cups sweet potato, baked or steamed and cubed

- 1/3 cup quinoa flakes or gluten free rolled oats

- 2 heaping tablespoon flax meal

- 2-3 tablespoon lime juice (to taste)

- 2 tablespoon low sodium tamari

- 1/4 cup cilantro, chopped

- Dash red pepper flakes (optional)

- Water as needed

Directions:

1. Preheat oven to 350 F.

2. Heat coconut oil in a large pan or wok. Sauté onion and ginger in 1 teaspoon coconut oil (or coconut oil spray) till soft and fragrant (about 5 minutes).

3. Add chickpeas and heat through.

4. Place the chickpeas, onion, and ginger in a food processor and add the sweet potato, quinoa flakes or oats, flax seed, lime juice, cilantro, tamari or coconut aminos, and dash of red pepper flakes, if using.

5. Pulse to combine, then run the motor and add some water until consistency is very thick but easy to mold.

6. Shape mixture into 4-6 burgers. Bake at 350 degrees for about 35 minutes, flipping in between.

Nutrition:

Calories: 232, Carbs: 4g ,Fat: 42g ,Protein: 10g

Raw Cauliflower Rice with Lemon, Mint, and Pistachios

Preparation time: 10 minutes

Cooking time: 25 minutes

Servings: 6

Ingredients:

- 5 cups raw cauliflower florets

- 1 oz pistachios

- 1/4 cup each basil and mint

- 2 teaspoon lemon zest

- 1-1/2 tablespoon lemon juice

- 1 tablespoon olive oil

- 1/4 cup dried currants

- Sea salt and black pepper to taste

Directions:

1. Transfer 3 cups of the cauliflower to a food processor.

2. Process until the cauliflower is broken down into pieces that are about the size of rice.

3. Transfer to a large mixing bowl.

4. Transfer remaining 2 cups of cauliflower to the food processor.

5. Add the pistachios and process, once again, until cauliflower is broken down into rice sized pieces.

6. Pulse in the basil and mint till herbs are finely chopped.

7. Add the additional chopped cauliflower, pistachios, and herbs to the mixing bowl with the first batch of cauliflower.

8. Add the lemon juice, oil, and currents.

9. Season to taste with salt and pepper and serve.

Nutrition:

Calories: 212

Carbs: 2g

Fat: 5g

Protein: 13g

Avocado Toast with Chickpeas

Preparation time: 5 minutes

Cooking time: 5 minutes

Servings: 2

Ingredients:

- 1/2 of avocado, peeled, pitted

- 4 tablespoons canned chickpeas, liquid reserved

- 1 tablespoon lime juice

- 1 teaspoon apple cider vinegar

- 2 slices of bread, toasted

- 1/4 teaspoon salt

- 1/4 teaspoon paprika

- 1 teaspoon olive oil

Directions:

1. Take a medium skillet pan, place it over medium heat, add oil and when hot, add chickpeas and cook for 2 minutes.

2. Sprinkle 1/8 teaspoon each salt and paprika over chickpeas, toss to coat, and then remove the pan from heat.

3. Place avocado in a bowl, mash by using a fork, drizzle with lime juice and vinegar and stir until well mixed.

4. Spread mashed avocado over bread slices, scatter chickpeas on top and then serve.

Nutrition:

Calories: 235

Carbs: 5g

Fat: 5g

Protein: 31g

Mashed Potatoes

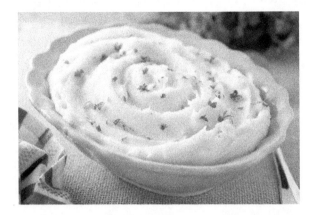

Preparation time: 10 minutes

Cooking time: 12 minutes

Servings: 2

Ingredients:

- 4 potatoes, halved

- 1/4 tablespoons chives, chopped

- 1 teaspoon minced garlic

- 3/4 teaspoon sea salt

- 2 tablespoons vegan butter, unsalted

- 1/4 teaspoon ground black pepper

Directions:

1. Take a medium pot, place it over medium-high heat, add potatoes, cover with water and boil until cooked and tender.

2. When done, drain the potatoes, let them cool for 10 minutes, peel them and return them into the pot.

3. Mash the potatoes by using a hand mixer until fluffy, add remaining **Ingredients:** except for chives, and then stir until mixed.

4. Sprinkle chives over the top and then serve.

Nutrition:

Calories: 365

Carbs: 10g

Fat: 5g

Protein: 67g

Green Onion Soup

Preparation time: 5 minutes

Cooking time: 12 minutes

Servings: 2

Ingredients:

- 6 green onions, chopped

- 7 ounces diced potatoes

- 1/3 teaspoon salt

- 2 tablespoons olive oil

- 1 1/4 cup vegetable broth

- 1/4 teaspoon ground white pepper

- 1/4 teaspoon ground coriander

Directions:

1. Take a small pan, place potato in it, cover with water, and then place the pan over medium heat.

2. Boil the potato until cooked and tender, and when done, drain the potatoes and set aside until required.

3. Return saucepan over low heat, add oil and add green onions and cook for 5 minutes until cooked.

4. Season with salt, pepper, and coriander, add potatoes, pour in vegetable broth, stir until mixed and bring it to simmer.

5. Then remove the pan from heat and blend the mixture by using an immersion blender until creamy.

6. Taste to adjust seasoning, then ladle soup into bowls and then serve.

Nutrition:

Calories: 191

Carbs: 1g

Fat: 1g

Protein: 15g

Broccoli Stir-Fry with Sesame Seeds

Preparation Time: 10 Minutes

Cooking Time: 8 Minutes

Servings: 4

Ingredients:

- Two tablespoons extra-virgin olive oil (optional)

- One tablespoon grated fresh ginger

- cups broccoli florets

- ¼ teaspoon sea salt (optional)

- Two garlic cloves, minced

- Two tablespoons toasted sesame seeds

Directions:

1. Heat the olive oil (if desired) in a large nonstick skillet over medium-high heat until shimmering.

2. Fold in the ginger, broccoli, and sea salt (if desired) and stir-fry for 5 to 7 minutes, or until the broccoli is browned.

3. Cook the garlic until tender, about 30 seconds.

4. Sprinkle with the sesame seeds and serve warm.

Nutrition:

calories: 135

fat: 10.9g

carbs: 9.7g

protein: 4.1g

fiber: 3.3g

Pasta & Noodles

Stir Fry Noodles

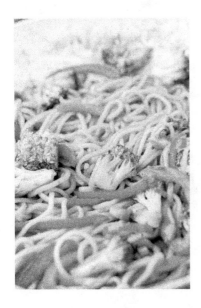

Preparation Time: 10 minutes

Cooking Time: 8 minutes

Servings: 4

Ingredients:

- 1 cup broccoli, chopped
- 1 cup red bell pepper, chopped
- 1 cup mushrooms, chopped
- 1 large onion, chopped

- 1 batch Stir Fry Sauce, prepared
- Salt and black pepper, to taste
- 2 cups spaghetti, cooked
- 4 garlic cloves, minced
- 2 tablespoons sesame oil

Directions:

1. Heat sesame oil in a pan over medium heat and add garlic, onions, bell pepper, broccoli, mushrooms.
2. Sauté for about 5 minutes and add spaghetti noodles and stir fry sauce.
3. Mix well and cook for 3 more minutes.
4. Dish out in plates and serve to enjoy.

Nutrition:

Calories: 567

Total Fat: 48g

Total Carbs: 6g

Fiber: 4g;

Net Carbs: 2g

Sodium: 373mg

Protein: 33g

Spicy Sweet Chili Veggie Noodles

Preparation Time: 10 minutes

Cooking Time: 7 minutes

Servings: 2

Ingredients:

- 1 head of broccoli, cut into bite sized florets
- 1 onion, finely sliced
- 1 tablespoon olive oil
- 1 courgette, halved
- 2 nests of whole-wheat noodles
- 150g mushrooms, sliced
- For Sauce
- 3 tablespoons soy sauce
- ¼ cup sweet chili sauce
- 1 teaspoon Sriracha
- 1 tablespoon peanut butter
- 2 tablespoons boiled water
- For Topping
- 2 teaspoons sesame seeds
- 2 teaspoons dried chili flakes

Directions:

1. Heat olive oil on medium heat in a saucepan and add onions.
2. Sauté for about 2 minutes and add broccoli, courgette and mushrooms.
3. Cook for about 5 minutes, stirring occasionally.
4. Whisk sweet chili sauce, soy sauce, Sriracha, water and peanut butter in a bowl.
5. Cook the noodles according to packet instructions and add to the vegetables.
6. Stir in the sauce and top with dried chili flakes and sesame seeds to serve.

Nutrition:

Calories: 351

Total Fat: 27g

Protein: 25g

Total Carbs: 2g

Fiber: 1g

Net Carbs: 1g

Creamy Vegan Mushroom Pasta

Preparation Time: 10 minutes

Cooking Time: 30 minutes

Servings: 6

Ingredients:

2 cups frozen peas, thawed

3 tablespoons flour, unbleached

3 cups almond breeze, unsweetened

1 tablespoon nutritional yeast

1/3 cup fresh parsley, chopped, plus extra for garnish

¼ cup olive oil

1 pound pasta of choice

4 cloves garlic, minced

2/3 cup shallots, chopped

8 cups mixed mushrooms, sliced

Salt and black pepper, to taste

Directions:

Take a bowl and boil pasta in salted water.

Heat olive oil in a pan over medium heat.

Add mushrooms, garlic, shallots and ½ tsp salt and cook
for 15 minutes.

Sprinkle flour on the vegetables and stir for a minute while
cooking.

Add almond beverage, stir constantly.

Let it simmer for 5 minutes and add pepper to it.

Cook for 3 more minutes and remove from heat.

Stir in nutritional yeast.

Add peas, salt, and pepper.

Cook for another minute and add

Add pasta to this sauce.

Garnish and serve!

Nutrition:

Calories: 364

Total Fat: 28g

Protein: 24g

Total Carbs: 4g

Fiber: 2g

Net Carbs: 2g

Vegan Chinese Noodles

Preparation Time: 15 minutes

Cooking Time: 8 minutes

Servings: 4

Ingredients:

- 300 g mixed oriental mushrooms, such as oyster, shiitake and enoki, cleaned and sliced
- 200 g thin rice noodles, cooked according to packet instructions and drained
- 2 garlic cloves, minced
- 1 fresh red chili
- 200 g courgettes, sliced
- 6 spring onions, reserving the green part
- 1 teaspoon corn flour
- 1 tablespoon agave syrup
- 1 teaspoon sesame oil
- 100 g baby spinach, chopped
- Hot chili sauce, to serve
- 2(1-inch) pieces of ginger
- ½ bunch fresh coriander, chopped
- 4 tablespoons vegetable oil
- 2 tablespoons low-salt soy sauce
- ½ tablespoon rice wine
- 2 limes, to serve

Directions:

Heat sesame oil over high heat in a large wok and add the mushrooms.

Sauté for about 4 minutes and add garlic, chili, ginger, courgette, coriander stalks and the white part of the spring onions.

Sauté for about 3 minutes until softened and lightly golden.

Meanwhile, combine the corn flour and 2 tablespoons of water in a bowl.

Add soy sauce, agave syrup, sesame oil and rice wine to the corn flour mixture.

Put this mixture in the pan to the veggie mixture and cook for about 3 minutes until thickened.

Add the spinach and noodles and mix well.

Stir in the coriander leaves and top with lime wedges, hot chili sauce and reserved spring onions to serve.

Nutrition:

Calories: 314,Total Fat: 22g,Protein: 26g,Total Carbs: 3g,Fiber: 0.3g,Net Carbs: 2.7g

Vegetable Penne Pasta

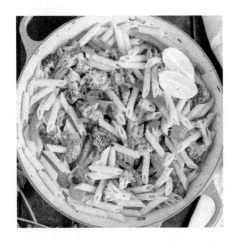

Preparation Time: 15 minutes

Cooking Time: 20 minutes

Servings: 6

Ingredients:

½ large onion, chopped

2 celery sticks, chopped

½ tablespoon ginger paste

½ cup green bell pepper

1½ tablespoons soy sauce

½ teaspoon parsley

Salt and black pepper, to taste

½ pound penne pasta, cooked

2 large carrots, diced

½ small leek, chopped

1 tablespoon olive oil

½ teaspoon garlic paste

½ tablespoon Worcester sauce

½ teaspoon coriander

1 cup water

Directions:

Heat olive oil in a wok on medium heat and add onions, garlic and ginger paste.

Sauté for about 3 minutes and stir in all bell pepper, celery sticks, carrots and leek.

Sauté for about 5 minutes and add remaining ingredients except for pasta.

Cover the lid and cook for about 12 minutes.

Stir in the cooked pasta and dish out to serve warm.

Nutrition:

Calories: 385

Total Fat: 29g

Protein: 26g

Total Carbs: 5g

Fiber: 1g

Net Carbs: 4g

Spaghetti in Spicy Tomato Sauce

Preparation Time: 15 minutes

Cooking Time: 40 minutes

Servings: 4

Ingredients:

- 1 pound dried spaghetti
- 1 red bell pepper, diced
- 4 garlic cloves, minced
- 1 teaspoon red pepper flakes, crushed
- 2 (14-ounce) cans diced tomatoes
- 1 (6-ounce) can tomato paste
- 2 teaspoons vegan sugar, granulated
- 2 tablespoons olive oil
- 1 medium onion, diced
- 1 cup dry red wine
- 1 teaspoon dried thyme
- ½ teaspoon fennel seed, crushed
- 1½ cups coconut milk, full-Fat
- Salt and black pepper, to taste

Directions:

Boil water in a large pot and add pasta.

Cook according to the package directions and drain the
pasta into a colander.

Dish out the pasta in a large serving bowl and add a dash of olive oil to prevent sticking.

Heat 2 tablespoons of olive oil over medium heat in a large pot and add garlic, onion and bell pepper.

Sauté for about 5 minutes and stir in the wine, thyme, fennel and red pepper flakes.

Allow to simmer on high heat for about 5 minutes until the liquid is reduced by about half.

Add diced tomatoes and tomato paste and allow to simmer for about 20 minutes, stirring occasionally.

Stir in the coconut milk and sugar and simmer for about 10 more minutes.

Season with salt and black pepper and pour the sauce over the pasta.

Toss to coat well and dish out in plates to serve.

Nutrition:

Calories: 313

Total Fat: 25g

Protein: 21g

Total Carbs: 1g

Fiber: 0g

Net Carbs: 1g

Bok Choy Stir-Fry

Preparation Time: 12 Minutes

Cooking Time: 10 to 13 Minutes

Servings: 4 to 6

Ingredients:

- Two tablespoons coconut oil (optional)

- One large onion, finely diced

- Two teaspoons ground cumin

- 1-inch piece fresh ginger, grated

- One teaspoon ground turmeric

- ½ teaspoon salt (optional)

- 12 baby bok choy heads, ends trimmed and sliced lengthwise

- Water, as needed

- cups cooked brown rice

Directions:

1. Heat the coconut oil (if desired) in a large pan over medium heat.

2. Sauté with onion for 5 minutes until translucent.

3. Stir in the cumin, ginger, turmeric, and salt (if desired). Combine the bok choy and stir-fry for 5 to 8 minutes or until the bok choy is tender but still crisp.

4. Pour water 1 to 2 tablespoons at a time to keep from sticking to the pan.

5. Serve over the brown rice.

Nutrition:

calories: 447

fat: 8.9g

carbs: 75.6g

protein: 29.7g

fiber: 19.1g

Creamy Vegan Pumpkin Pasta

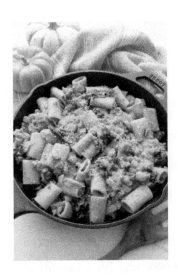

Preparation Time: 15 minutes

Cooking Time: 5 minutes

Servings: 6

Ingredients:

  1 tablespoon olive oil

  1 cup raw cashews, soaked in water 4-8 hours, drained and
     rinsed

  12 ounces dried penne pasta

  1 cup pumpkin puree, canned

  1 cup almond milk, plus more as needed

  3 garlic cloves

  ¼ teaspoon ground nutmeg

Fresh parsley, for garnish

1 tablespoon lemon juice

¾ teaspoon salt

1 tablespoon fresh sage, chopped

Directions:

Boil salted water in a large pot and add pasta.

Cook according to the package directions and drain the pasta into a colander.

Dish out the pasta in a large serving bowl and add a dash of olive oil to prevent sticking.

Put the pumpkin, cashews, milk, lemon juice, garlic, salt and nutmeg into the food processor and blend until smooth.

Stir in the sauce and sage over the pasta and toss to coat well.

Garnish with fresh parsley and dish out to serve hot.

NUTRITION:

Calories: 431

Total Fat: 31g

Protein: 35g

Total Carbs: 3g

Fiber: 0.5g

Net Carbs: 2.5g

Loaded Creamy Vegan Pesto Pasta

Preparation Time: 15 minutes

Cooking Time: 10 minutes

Servings: 6

Ingredients:

  ¼ onion, finely chopped

  8 romaine lettuce leaves

  1 celery stalk, thinly sliced

  ½ cup blue cheese, crumbled

  1 tablespoon olive oil, plus a dash

  1 cup almond milk, unflavored and unsweetened

  ½ cup vegan pesto

  1 cup chickpeas, cooked

  1 cup fresh arugula, packed

  2 tablespoons lemon juice

  Salt and black pepper, to taste

  6-ounces orecchiette pasta, dried

  1 cup full-Fat coconut milk

  2 tablespoons whole wheat flour

  1½ cups cherry tomatoes, halved

  ½ cup Kalamata olives, halved

  Red pepper flakes, to taste

Directions:

Boil salted water in a large pot and add pasta.

Cook according to the package directions and drain the pasta into a colander.

Dish out the pasta in a large serving bowl and add a dash of olive oil to prevent sticking.

Put olive oil over medium heat in a large pot and whisk in the flour.

Cook for about 4 minutes, until the mixture begins to smell nutty and stir in the coconut milk and almond milk.

Let the sauce simmer for about 1 minute and add the chickpeas, olives and arugula.

Stir well and season with lemon juice, red pepper flakes, and salt and black pepper.

Dish out into plates and serve hot.

Nutrition:

Calories: 220

Total Fat: 10g

Protein: 31g

Total Carbs: 1.5g

Fiber: 0.5g

Net Carbs: 1g

Creamy Vegan Spinach Pasta

Preparation Time: 20 minutes

Cooking Time: 5 minutes

Servings: 4

Ingredients:

1 cup raw cashews, soaked in water for 8 hours

2 tablespoons lemon juice

1 tablespoon olive oil

1½ cups vegetable broth

2 tablespoons fresh dill, chopped

Red pepper flakes, to taste

10 ounces dried fusilli

½ cup almond milk, unflavored and unsweetened

2 tablespoons white miso paste

4 garlic cloves, divided

8-ounces fresh spinach, finely chopped

¼ cup scallions, chopped

Salt and black pepper, to taste

Directions:

Boil salted water in a large pot and add pasta.

Cook according to the package directions and drain the
pasta into a colander.

Dish out the pasta in a large serving bowl and add a dash of
olive oil to prevent sticking.

Put the cashews, milk, miso, lemon juice, and 1 garlic clove
into the food processor and blend until smooth.

Put olive oil over medium heat in a large pot and add the
remaining 3 cloves of garlic.

Sauté for about 1 minute and stir in the spinach and broth.

Raise the heat and allow to simmer for about 4 minutes
until the spinach is bright green and wilted.

Stir in the pasta and cashew mixture and season with salt
and black pepper.

Top with scallions and dill and dish out into plates to serve.

Nutrition:

Calories: 94

Total Fat: 10g

Protein: 0g

Total Carbs: 1g

Fiber: 0.3g

Net Carbs: 0.7g

Vegan Bake Pasta with Bolognese Sauce and Cashew Cream

Preparation Time: 1 hour 10 minutes

Cooking Time: 20 minutes

Servings: 8

Ingredients:

For the Pasta:

    1 packet penne pasta

For the Bolognese Sauce:

    1 tablespoon soy sauce

    1 small can lentils

    1 tablespoon brown sugar

    ½ cup tomato paste

    1 teaspoon garlic, crushed

    1 tablespoon olive oil

    2 tomatoes, chopped

    1 onion, chopped

    2 cups mushrooms, sliced

    Salt, to taste

    Pepper, to taste

    For the Cashew Cream:

    1 cup raw cashews

    ½ lemon, squeezed

½ teaspoon salt

½ cup water

For the White Sauce:

1 teaspoon black pepper

1 teaspoon Dijon mustard

¼ cup nutritional yeast

Sea salt, as required

2 cups coconut milk

3 tablespoons vegan butter

2 tablespoons all-purpose flour

1/3 cup vegetable broth

Directions:

Take a pot and boil water, add pasta to it, boil for 3 minutes
and set aside.

Fry onion and garlic, mushroom in olive oil and add soy
sauce to it.

Add in sugar tomato paste, lentils, and canned tomato to it
and let it simmer, Bolognese sauce is prepared.

Season it with salt and black pepper.

Add the lemon juice, cashews, water and salt to the blender,
blend for 2 minutes.

Add this to the sauce you have prepared and stir pasta in it.

Melt the vegan butter in a saucepan, add in the flour and
stir.

Add vegetable stock and coconut milk to it and whisk well.

Stir continuously and let it boil for about 5 minutes, then remove from heat.

Add Dijon mustard, nutritional yeast, black pepper, and sea salt.

Preheat the oven to 430 degrees F.

Prepare rectangular oven-safe dish by placing pasta and Bolognese sauce to it.

Pour the white sauce on it and bake for a time period of 20-25 minutes.

Nutrition:

Calories: 314

Total Fat: 20g

Protein: 31g

Total Carbs: 2.5g

Fiber: 0.8g

Net Carbs: 1.7g

Asian Veggie Noodles

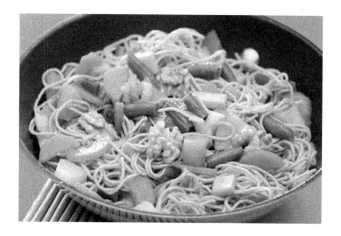

Preparation Time: 10 minutes

Cooking Time: 20 minutes

Servings: 4

Ingredients:

½ cup peas

1 teaspoon rice vinegar

3 carrots, chopped

1 small packet vermicelli

3 tablespoons sesame oil

1 red pepper, chopped in small cubes

1 can baby corn

1 clove garlic, chopped

2 tablespoons soy sauce

1 teaspoon ginger powder

½ teaspoon curry powder

Salt and black pepper, to taste

Directions:

Take a bowl and add ginger powder, vinegar, soy sauce, curry powder, and a pinch of salt to it.

Cook the noodles according to the instructions and drain them.

Heat the sesame oil and cook vegetables in it for 10 minutes on medium heat.

Add noodles to it and cook for 3 more minutes.

Remove from heat and serve to enjoy.

Nutrition:

Calories: 329

Total Fat: 25g

Protein: 20g

Total Carbs: 6g

Fiber: 1g

Net Carbs: 5g

Plant Based Keto Lo Mein

Preparation Time: 10 Minutes

Cooking Time: 10 Minutes

Serving: 2

Ingredients:

2 tablespoons carrots, shredded

1 package kelp noodles, soaked in water

1 cup broccoli, frozen

For the Sauce

1 tablespoon sesame oil

2 tablespoons tamari

1/2 teaspoon ground ginger

1/4 teaspoon Sriracha

1/2 teaspoon garlic powder

Directions:

Put the broccoli in a saucepan on medium low heat and add the sauce **Ingredients:**.

Cook for about 5 minutes and add the noodles after draining water.

Allow to simmer about 10 minutes, occasionally stirring to avoid burning.

When the noodles have softened, mix everything well and dish out to serve.

Nutrition:

Calories: 97

Net Carbs: 2.1g

Fat: 7g

Carbohydrates: 6.2g

Fiber: 2.1g

Sugar: 1.6g

Protein: 3.4g

Sodium: 1047mg

Vegetarian Chowmein

Preparation Time: 20 Minutes

Cooking Time: 30 Minutes

Serving: 2

Ingredients:

1/2 large onion, chopped

1/2 small leek, chopped

1/2 tablespoon ginger paste

1/2 tablespoon Worcester sauce

1/2 tablespoon Oriental seasoning

1/2 teaspoon parsley

Salt and black pepper, to taste

1/2 pound noodles

2 large carrots, diced

2 celery sticks, chopped

1 tablespoon olive oil

1/2 teaspoon garlic paste

11/2 tablespoons soy sauce

1 tablespoon Chinese five spice

1/2 teaspoon coriander

2 cups water

Directions:

Put olive oil, ginger, garlic paste, and onion in a pot on
medium heat and sauté for about 5 minutes.

Stir in all the vegetables and cook for about5 minutes.

Add rest of the **Ingredients:** and combine well.

Secure the lid and cook on medium heat for about 20
minutes, stirring occasionally.

Open the lid and dish out to serve hot.

Nutrition:

Calories: 334

Net Carbs: 41.1g

Fat: 11.7g

Carbohydrates: 48.9g

Fiber: 5.2g

Sugar: 7.1g

Protein: 9.7g

Sodium: 807mg

Conclusion

In a nutshell, this cookbook offers you a world full of options to diversify your plant-based menu. People on this diet are usually seen struggling to choose between healthy food and flavor but, soon, they run out of the options. The selection of 250 recipes in this book is enough to adorn your dinner table with flavorsome, plant-based meals every day. Give each recipe a good read and try them out in the kitchen. You will experience tempting aromas and binding flavors every day.

The book is conceptualized with the idea of offering you a comprehensive view of a plant-based diet and how it can benefit the body. You may find the shift sudden, especially if you are a die-hard fan of non-vegetarian items. But you need not give up anything that you love. Eat everything in moderation.

The next step is to start experimenting with the different recipes in this book and see which ones are your favorites. Everyone has their favorite food, and you will surely find several of yours in this book. Start with breakfast and work your way through. You will be pleasantly surprised at how tasty a vegan meal really can be.

You will love reading this book, as it helps you to understand how revolutionary a plant-based diet can be. It will help you to make informed decisions as you move toward greater change for the greater good. What are you waiting for? Have you begun your journey on the path of the plant-based diet yet? If you haven't, do it now!

Now you have everything you need to get started making budget-friendly, healthy plant-based recipes. Just follow your basic shopping list and follow your meal plan to get started! It's easy to switch over to a plant-based diet if you have your meals planned out and temptation locked away. Don't forget to clean out your kitchen before starting, and you're sure to meet all your diet and health goals.

You need to plan if you are thinking about dieting. First, you can start slowly by just eating one meal a day, which is vegetarian and gradually increasing your number of vegetarian meals. Whenever you are struggling, ask your friend or family member to support you and keep you motivated. One important thing is also to be regularly accountable for not following the diet.

If dieting seems very important to you and you need to do it right, then it is recommended that you visit a professional such as a nutritionist or dietitian to discuss your dieting plan and optimizing it for the better.